The Slow Cooker Healthy Recipe book

Tasty and Delicious Side Dishes to Enjoy Your meals

Donna Conway

© copyright 2021 – all rights reserved.

the content contained within this book may not be reproduced, duplicated or transmitted without direct written permission from the author or the publisher.

under no circumstances will any blame or legal responsibility be held against the publisher, or author, for any damages, reparation, or monetary loss due to the information contained within this book. either directly or indirectly.

legal notice:

this book is copyright protected. this book is only for personal use. you cannot amend, distribute, sell, use, quote or paraphrase any part, or the content within this book, without the consent of the author or publisher.

disclaimer notice:

please note the information contained within this document is for educational and entertainment purposes only. all effort has been executed to present accurate, up to date, and reliable, complete information. no warranties of any kind are declared or implied. readers acknowledge that the author is not engaging in the rendering of legal, financial, medical or professional advice. the content within this book has been derived from various sources. please consult a licensed professional before attempting any techniques outlined in this book.

by reading this document, the reader agrees that under no circumstances is the author responsible for any losses, direct or indirect, which are incurred as a result of the use of information contained within this document, including, but not limited to, — errors, omissions, or inaccuracies.

Table of Contents

- BAKED BEANS 6
- BBQ BEANS 8
- SWEET & TANGY COWBOY BEANS 10
- JALAPENO PINTO BEANS 12
- HAWAIIAN BEANS 14
- HEALTHY WILD RICE 16
- HERBED BROWN RICE 18
- RED BEANS & RICE 20
- PUMPKIN RISOTTO 22
- PARMESAN RISOTTO 24
- MEXICAN RICE 26
- MEXICAN QUINOA 28
- APPLE CINNAMON QUINOA 30
- SPINACH BARLEY RISOTTO 32
- CUBAN BLACK BEANS 33
- TOMATILLO RICE 35
- VEGETABLE FRIED RICE 37
- PAELLA 39
- PORTOBELLO BARLEY 41
- WILD RICE WITH MIXED VEGETABLES 43
- SAFFRON RICE 44
- BULGUR WITH BROCCOLI AND CARROT 45
- RED BEANS AND RICE 46
- SPINACH RICE 48
- BROWN RICE AND VEGETABLES 50
- CURRIED RICE 52
- CHIPOTLE BLACK BEAN SALAD 54

Mediterranean Chickpeas	56
Curried Lentils	58
Bourbon Baked Beans	60
Italian Chickpeas	62
Sweet and Spicy Chickpeas	64
Mediterranean Chickpeas and Brown Rice	66
Rice Pilaf	68
Wild Rice and Mushroom Casserole	69
Rice with Chicken and Asparagus	71
Cilantro-Lime Chicken and Rice	73
Indian Spiced Brown Rice with Ground Lamb	75
Barley and Chickpea Risotto	77
Coconut Quinoa Curry	79
Sweet and Sour Beans	81
Navy Bean Soup with Ham	83
Coconut Red Beans and Rice	85
Ranch Style Pinto Beans	87
Garlic Veggie Lentils	89
Vegetarian Calico Beans	91
Summer Squash Mix	93
Hot Zucchini Mix	95
Creamy Butter Parsnips	97
Butternut Squash and Eggplant Mix	99
Classic Veggies Mix	101
Spinach and Squash Side Salad	103
Cheddar Potatoes Mix	105
Okra and Corn	107

Baked Beans

Preparation time: 10 minutes

Cooking time: 8 hours

Serve: 4 people

Ingredients:

- 3 cups dried navy beans, soaked in water overnight & drained
- 4 cups chicken broth
- 1/4 cup molasses
- 3/4 cup brown sugar
- 15 oz can tomato sauce
- 1/4 tsp cayenne pepper
- 1 tsp black pepper
- 1 tbsp ground mustard
- 1 bell pepper, diced
- 1 onion, diced
- 1 lb. bacon, cut into 1-inch pieces

- 1 tbsp kosher salt

Directions:

1. Add bacon, bell pepper, and onion into the slow cooker. Sauté until onion softens. Add remaining ingredients into it and stir well. Cook on low for 8 hours. Stir and serve.

Nutrition:

Calories: 561

Fat: 20.9g

Carbs: 60.5g

Protein: 33.8g

BBQ Beans

Preparation time: 10 minutes

Cooking time: 6 hours

Serving: 4 people

Ingredients:

- 15 oz can kidney beans, drained & rinsed
- 30 oz can great northern beans, drained & rinsed
- 30 oz can black beans, drained & rinsed
- 2 lbs. kielbasa, cut into bite-size pieces
- 1/2 lb. bacon, cooked & chopped
- 14 oz chicken broth
- 1/4 cup molasses
- 1/2 cup maple syrup
- 1 tbsp apple cider vinegar
- 1 tsp chili powder
- 1 tbsp mustard
- 1 tbsp Worcestershire sauce

- 3/4 cup ketchup
- 1/2 cup BBQ sauce
- 1 onion, diced

Directions:

1. Add all ingredients except kielbasa into the slow cooker and stir well. Top with kielbasa and stir gently. Cook on low for 6 hours. Stir and serve.

Nutrition:

Calories: 412

Fat: 16.9g

Carbs: 44.5g

Protein: 21.8g

Sweet & Tangy Cowboy Beans

Preparation time: 10 minutes

Cooking time: 4 hours

Servings: 4 people

Ingredients:

- 1 lb. ground beef
- 15 oz can pork and beans
- 15 oz can white beans
- 15 oz of kidney beans
- 2 tbsp bacon drippings
- 1 lb. bacon, cooked and chopped
- 2 1/2 tbsp yellow mustard
- 1/4 cup molasses
- 1 cup ketchup
- 3/4 cup brown sugar
- 1 large onion, diced

Directions:

1. Add ground beef and onion into the slow cooker and sauté until meat is no longer pink. Add remaining fixing into the slow cooker and stir well. Cook on high for 4 hours. Stir and serve.

Nutrition:

Calories: 279

Fat: 11.8g

Carbs: 24.6g

Protein: 19.7g

Jalapeno Pinto Beans

Preparation time: 10 minutes

Cooking time: 8 hours

Servings: 4 people

Ingredients:

- 1 lb. pinto beans, soak in water for overnight & drain
- 14 oz beef broth
- 32 oz vegetable broth
- 6 bacon sliced, cooked & chopped
- 2 jalapeno peppers, seeded & chopped
- 15 oz can tomato, diced & drained
- 1 tsp garlic powder
- 1 tsp cumin
- 1 tsp black pepper
- 1 tbsp garlic, minced
- 1 onion, sliced

Directions:

1. Add all fixing into the slow cooker and stir well. Cook on high for 8 hours. Stir and serve.

Nutrition:

Calories: 441

Fat: 5.4g

Carbs: 55g

Protein: 30.8g

Hawaiian Beans

Preparation time: 10 minutes

Cooking time: 8 hours

Servings: 4 people

Ingredients:

- 15 oz kidney beans, rinsed & drained
- 15 oz white beans, rinsed & drained
- 28 oz pinto beans, rinsed & drained
- 1 tbsp Cajun seasoning
- 6 oz pineapple juice
- 1 tbsp Worcestershire sauce
- 2 tbsp Dijon mustard
- 2 tbsp vinegar
- 1/3 cup molasses
- 1/3 cup brown sugar
- 1/2 cup ketchup
- 1 tbsp garlic, minced

- 1/2 onion, diced

Directions:

1. Add all fixing into the slow cooker and stir well. Cook on low for 8 hours. Stir and serve.

Nutrition:

Calories: 187

Fat: 0.9g

Carbs: 39.1g

Protein: 8.2g

Healthy Wild Rice

Preparation time: 10 minutes

Cooking time: 6 hours

Servings: 4 people

Ingredients:

- 12 oz wild rice
- 8 oz mushrooms, sliced
- 21 oz vegetable broth
- 1/4 cup pecans, chopped
- 1/8 tsp black pepper
- 1/2 tsp dried tarragon
- 1/2 tsp dried marjoram
- 1/3 cup onion, diced
- 3 tbsp soy sauce
- 1 tbsp butter
- 1/2 cup carrot, chopped
- 1 tsp sea salt

Directions:

1. Add all ingredients except pecans into the slow cooker and stir well. Cook on low for 6 hours. Add pecans and mix well and let it sit for 10 minutes. Stir and serve.

Nutrition:

Calories: 434

Fat: 10.2g

Carbs: 70.5g

Protein: 19.2g

Herbed Brown Rice

Preparation time: 10 minutes

Cooking time: 3 hours

Servings: 4 people

Ingredients:

- 2 cups brown rice
- 1/2 tsp dried oregano
- 1/2 tsp dried thyme
- 4 cups chicken broth
- 8 oz mushrooms, sliced
- 2 tbsp butter
- Pepper
- salt

Directions:

1. Add butter into the slow cooker and set on sauté mode. Once butter is melted, add brown rice into the slow cooker and sauté for 2-4 minutes.

2. Add the rest of the fixing into the slow cooker and stir well—cook on high for 3 hours. Stir well and serve.

Nutrition:

Calories: 446

Fat: 9.9g

Carbs: 75.4g

Protein: 13.9g

Red Beans & Rice

Preparation time: 10 minutes

Cooking time: 8 hours

Servings: 4 people

Ingredients:

- 2 cups dried red beans, soaked & drained
- 4 cups of water
- 1/2 lb. smoked sausage, cut into small pieces
- 2 garlic cloves, minced
- 1/2 cup onion, chopped
- Pepper
- Salt

Directions:

1. Add all fixing into the slow cooker and stir well. Cook on low for 7 hours and 30 minutes. Remove 1/4 cup beans from the slow cooker and mash well. Return mashed beans into the slow cooker and cook for 30 minutes more. Stir and serve.

Nutrition:

Calories: 340

Fat: 11.4g

Carbs: 38.8g

Protein: 21.3g

Pumpkin Risotto

Preparation time: 10 minutes

Cooking time: 1 hour 30 minutes

Servings: 4 people

Ingredients:

- 1 1/2 cup Arborio rice
- 2 cups roasted pumpkin
- 1 tsp black pepper
- 4 cups vegetable broth
- 1/2 cup onion, chopped
- 1 tbsp garlic, crushed
- 2 tsp dried sage
- 2 tbsp olive oil
- 2 tsp salt

Directions:

1. Add oil into the slow cooker and set on sauté mode. Add onion, garlic, and sage into the slow cooker and sauté until onion is softened.

2. Add remaining fixing into the slow cooker and stir well. Cook on high for 1 hour and 30 minutes. Stir well and serve.

Nutrition:

Calories: 509

Fat: 15g

Carbs: 77.4g

Protein: 15.9g

Parmesan Risotto

Preparation time: 10 minutes

Cooking time: 2 hours

Servings: 6 people

Ingredients:

- 1 1/4 cups Arborio rice
- 3/4 cup parmesan cheese, shredded
- 1 tbsp garlic powder
- 1 tbsp dried onion flakes
- 1/4 cup white wine
- 1/4 cup olive oil
- 4 cups vegetable broth
- 1/2 tsp black pepper
- 1 tsp kosher salt

Directions:

1. Add all ingredients except parmesan cheese into the slow cooker and stir well. Cook on high for 2 hours. Add parmesan cheese and mix well. Serve and enjoy.

Nutrition:

Calories: 351

Fat: 15.8g

Carbs: 35.2g

Protein: 15.6g

Mexican Rice

Preparation time: 10 minutes

Cooking time: 5 hours

Servings: 4 people

Ingredients:

- 1 cup white rice
- 1/2 tsp dried oregano
- 1/2 tsp chili powder
- 1 tsp cumin
- 1/4 tsp black pepper
- 1/2 jalapeno, chopped
- 4 oz can green chilies, diced
- 1/2 cup can tomato, diced
- 1 cup tomato sauce
- 1 cup chicken stock
- 1/2 tsp salt

Directions:

1. Add all fixing into the slow cooker and stir well. Cook on low for 5 hours. Stir well and serve.

Nutrition:

Calories: 203

Fat: 0.9g

Carbs: 44g

Protein: 4.9g

Mexican Quinoa

Preparation time: 10 minutes

Cooking time: 2 hours

Servings: 4 people

Ingredients:

- 3/4 cup quinoa, rinsed
- 14 oz black beans, rinsed & drained
- 1/2 tsp garlic, minced
- 1 tsp cumin
- 1 bay leaf
- 3/4 cup salsa
- 1 1/2 cups water
- 1 tsp salt

Directions:

1. Add all fixing into the slow cooker and stir well. Cook on high for 2 hours. Fluff quinoa with fork and discard bay leaf. Stir well and serve.

Nutrition:

Calories: 150

Fat: 1.7g

Carbs: 27.7g

Protein: 7.1g

Apple Cinnamon Quinoa

Preparation time: 10 minutes

Cooking time: 2 hours

Servings: 4 people

Ingredients:

- 1 cup quinoa, rinsed
- 1 tsp vanilla
- 1/4 tsp nutmeg
- 2 tsp cinnamon
- 1 apple, peel & dice
- 1/4 cup pepitas
- 4 dates, chopped
- 3 cups almond milk
- 1/4 tsp salt

Directions:

1. Add all fixing into the slow cooker and stir well. Cook on high for 2 hours. Stir well and serve.

Nutrition:

Calories: 504

Fat: 37.2g

Carbs: 42.1g

Protein: 8.8g

Spinach Barley Risotto

Preparation time: 10 minutes

Cooking time: 6 hours

Servings: 4 people

Ingredients:

- 1 cup pearl barley
- 1/2 cup halloumi, cut into small pieces
- 2 1/2 cups fresh spinach, chopped
- 2 1/2 cups vegetable stock
- 2 garlic cloves, chopped
- 1 onion, chopped

Directions:

1. Add barley, stock, garlic, and onion into the slow cooker and stir well. Cook on low for 6 hours. Put the spinach and stir until spinach is wilted. Top with halloumi and serve.

Nutrition: Calories: 237, Fat: 3.9g, Carbs: 43.6g, Protein: 8.8g

Cuban Black Beans

Preparation time: 10 minutes

Cooking time: 8 hours

Servings: 4 people

Ingredients:

- 16 oz dry black beans, soak in water for overnight & drained
- 1 bay leaf
- 1 tomato, chopped
- 1 tsp balsamic vinegar
- 1/2 cup onion, diced
- 1/2 cup bell pepper, chopped
- 2 tbsp olive oil
- 2 garlic cloves, minced
- 1 tsp dry oregano
- 4 cups of water
- 1 tbsp salt

Directions:

1. Add oil into the slow cooker and set on sauté mode. Add onion, bell pepper, and garlic and sauté until onion is softened. Add remaining fixing into the slow cooker and stir well. Cook on low for 8 hours. Stir well and serve.

Nutrition:

Calories: 232

Fat: 4.4g

Carbs: 37.3g

Protein: 12.6 g

Tomatillo Rice

Preparation time: 15 minutes

Cooking time: 6 hours

Servings: 4 people

Ingredients:

- 2 tbsps. olive oil
- ½ red onion, diced
- ½ red bell pepper, diced
- 2 cloves garlic, minced
- Juice of 1 lime
- 1 cup tomatillo salsa
- 1 cup of water
- 1 tsp. salt
- 1 cup long-grain white rice
- ½ cup cilantro, chopped

Directions:

1. Heat oil in the slow cooker, then put the bell pepper, onion, and garlic and cook for 5 minutes. Add the rest of the fixing, except for the cilantro. Cover and cook on low within 6 hours. Stir in cilantro and serve.

Nutrition:

Calories: 268

Carbs: 47g

Fat: 7g

Protein: 5g

Vegetable Fried Rice

Preparation time: 15 minutes

Cooking time: 4 hours & 30 minutes

Servings: 4 people

Ingredients:

- 1 tbsp. butter
- 2 cups white rice, uncooked
- 3 garlic cloves, minced
- 2 cups of water
- 2 cups vegetable broth
- 2 ½ tsp soy sauce
- 1 tsp. brown sugar
- ½ tsp. Sriracha sauce
- 1 tsp. lime juice
- 1 cup carrots, diced
- 1 cup broccoli, chopped
- 1 egg, lightly beaten

Directions:

1. Grease the slow cooker with the butter. Add the rest of the fixing except for the egg. Cover and cook within 4 hours on low. Open and add the egg and cook for 30 minutes more.

Nutrition:

Calories: 390

Carbs: 70g

Fat: 3.6g

Protein: 9g

Paella

Preparation time: 15 minutes

Cooking time: 4 hours & 30 minutes

Servings: 4 people

Ingredients:

- 1 tbsp. butter
- ½ onion, diced
- 1 cup diced tomato
- ½ tsp. turmeric
- 1 tsp. salt
- 2 tbsp. fresh parsley
- 1 cup long-grain white rice
- 1 cup frozen peas
- 2 cups of water
- 1 (12-ounce) package vegan chorizo, crumbled

Directions:

1. Melt the butter in a slow cooker. Add onion and cook for 3 minutes. Add tomato, turmeric, salt, and parsley and mix. Add the rice, peas, and water.
2. Cover and cook on low within 4 hours. Pour the crumbled chorizo on top. Cover and cook for 30 minutes more. Serve.

Nutrition:

Calories: 421

Carbs: 32g

Fat: 24g

Protein: 17g

Portobello Barley

Preparation time: 15 minutes

Cooking time: 8 hours

Servings: 4 people

Ingredients:

- 1 tsp. olive oil
- 2 shallots, minced
- 2 cloves garlic, minced
- 3 portobello mushroom caps, sliced
- 1 cup pearl barley
- 3¼ cups water
- ¼ tsp. salt
- ½ tsp. freshly ground black pepper
- 1 tsp. crushed rosemary
- 1 tsp. dried chervil
- ¼ cup grated parmesan

Directions:

1. Heat oil on the slow cooker. Cook shallots, garlic, and mushrooms for 4 minutes. Add everything except for the parmesan. Cover and cook on low within 8 hours. Open and sprinkle with parmesan. Serve.

Nutrition:

Calories: 130

Carbs: 25g

Fat: 1.5g

Protein: 5g

Wild Rice with Mixed Vegetables

Preparation time: 15 minutes

Cooking time: 4 hours & 30 minutes

Servings: 4 people

Ingredients:

- 2½ cups water
- 1 cup wild rice
- 3 cloves garlic, minced
- 1 medium onion, diced
- 1 carrot, diced
- 1 stalk celery, diced

Directions:

1. Place all the fixings in the slow cooker and mix. Cover and cook on low for 4 hours. Then check if the kernels are open and tender. If not, then cover and cook for 15 to 30 minutes more. Serve.

Nutrition: Calories: 90, Carbs: 18g, Fat: 0g, Protein: 3

Saffron Rice

Preparation time: 15 minutes

Cooking time: 4 hours & 30 minutes

Servings: 4 people

Ingredients:

- 2 cups white rice, uncooked
- 2 tbsps. margarine
- 2 cups of water
- 2 cups vegetarian stock
- ¾ tsp. saffron threads
- 1 tsp. salt

Directions:

1. Add everything to the slow cooker. Cook on low for 4 hours. Check if the rice is tender. If not, then cook for 30 minutes more. Serve.

Nutrition: Calories: 420 Carbs: 82g Fat: 7g Protein: 9g

Bulgur with Broccoli and Carrot

Preparation time: 15 minutes

Cooking time: 7 hours

Servings: 4 people

Ingredients:

- 2 cups bulgur, uncooked
- 2 tbsps. butter
- 1 cup carrots, diced
- 1 cup broccoli, chopped
- 2 cups vegetable broth
- 1 tsp. salt

Directions:

1. Add everything to the slow cooker and cover. Cook on low for 6 hours. Check if it is tender; if not, cook for 1 hour more. Serve.

Nutrition: Calories: 360 Carbs: 13g Fat: 6g Protein: 9g

Red Beans and Rice

Preparation time: 15 minutes

Cooking time: 7 hours

Servings: 4 people

Ingredients:

- 3 cups of water
- 3½ cups vegetarian stock
- 2 tbsps. butter
- 1 can kidney beans, drained
- 2 cups white rice, uncooked
- 1 onion, chopped
- 1 green bell pepper, chopped
- 1 cup celery, chopped
- 1 tsp thyme
- 1 tsp paprika
- 1 tsp Cajun seasoning
- ½ tsp red pepper flakes

- 1 tsp salt
- ¼ tsp black pepper

Directions:

1. Add everything to the slow cooker. Cover and cook on low within 6 hours. Check the rice and cook 1 hour more if necessary. Serve.

Nutrition:

Calories: 340

Carbs: 52g

Fat: 7g

Protein: 11g

Spinach Rice

Preparation time: 15 minutes

Cooking time: 5 hours

Servings: 4 people

Ingredients:

- 2 cups spinach
- 2 cups white rice, uncooked
- 2 tbsps. butter
- 2 cups of water
- 2 cups vegetable broth
- 1 onion, diced
- 1 green bell pepper, diced
- 1 cup canned tomatoes, diced
- 1/8 cup pickled jalapenos, diced
- 1 tsp. chili powder
- ½ tsp. garlic powder
- 1 tsp. salt

- ¼ tsp. black pepper

Directions:

1. Add everything to the slow cooker. Cover and cook on low within 5 hours. Open and add the spinach. Cover and cook on Sauté for 5 minutes. Serve.

Nutrition:

Calories: 230

Carbs: 45g

Fat: 3g

Protein: 4g

Brown Rice and Vegetables

Preparation time: 15 minutes

Cooking time: 5 hours

Servings: 4 people

Ingredients:

- 2 cups brown rice, uncooked
- 2 tbsps. butter
- 3 cups vegetable broth
- 2 cups of water
- ½ cup yellow squash, chopped
- ½ cup zucchini, chopped
- ½ onion, chopped
- ½ cup button mushrooms, sliced
- ½ cup red bell pepper, chopped
- 1 tsp. salt
- ¼ tsp. black pepper

Directions:

1. Add everything to the slow cooker. Cover and cook on low within 5 hours. Serve.

Nutrition:

Calories: 225

Carbs: 42g

Fat: 4g

Protein: 4.6g

Curried Rice

Preparation time: 15 minutes

Cooking time: 4 hours & 30 minutes

Servings: 4 people

Ingredients:

- 2 cups white rice, uncooked
- 2 tbsp olive oil
- 2 cups of water
- 2 cups vegetable broth
- 2 tbsp curry powder
- 1 tsp salt
- ¼ tsp black pepper
- 1 tbsp lime juice
- ¼ cup cilantro, chopped

Directions:

1. Add all the fixings to the slow cooker except the lime juice and cilantro. Cover and cook on low within 4

hours. Stir in lime juice and cilantro and cook for 30 minutes more. Serve.

Nutrition:

Calories: 387

Carbs: 85g

Fat: 1g

Protein: 7.6g

Chipotle Black Bean Salad

Preparation time: 15 minutes

Cooking time: 5 hours

Servings: 4 people

Ingredients:

- 1 (16-ounce) bag dried black beans, soaked overnight and boiled for 10 minutes
- Enough water to cover beans by 1-inch
- 2 tsp salt
- 1 tbs. chipotle powder
- 2 tsp thyme
- 2 fresh tomatoes, diced
- 1 red onion, diced
- ¼ cup cilantro, chopped

Directions:

1. Put the black beans, water, plus salt in the slow cooker. Cover and cook on medium heat within 5

hours. Check the beans after 5 hours and cook 1 hour more if necessary. Drain the beans and cool. Mix in the remaining ingredients and serve.

Nutrition:

Calories: 198

Carbs: 37g

Fat: 1g

Protein: 10g

Mediterranean Chickpeas

Preparation time: 15 minutes

Cooking time: 2 hours

Servings: 4 people

Ingredients:

- 2 (15-ounce) cans chickpeas, drained
- 1 cup of water
- 4 tsp salt
- ¼ cup extra-virgin olive oil
- 1 tsp. black pepper
- 1 cup fresh basil, chopped
- 5 cloves garlic, minced
- 2 tomatoes, diced
- ½ cup kalamata olives, sliced

Directions:

1. Add everything in the slow cooker. Cover and cook on low within 2 hours. Serve.

Nutrition:

Calories: 243

Carbs: 37g

Fat: 8g

Protein: 7g

Curried Lentils

Preparation time: 15 minutes

Cooking time: 3 hours

Servings: 4 people

Ingredients:

- 2 tsp butter
- 1 large onion, thinly sliced
- 2 cloves garlic, minced
- 2 jalapenos, diced
- ½ tsp red pepper flakes
- ½ tsp ground cumin
- 1-pound yellow lentils
- 6 cups of water
- ½ tsp. salt
- ½ tsp. ground turmeric
- 4 cups chopped fresh spinach

Directions:

1. Melt the butter in a slow cooker. Cook the onions within 8 minutes or until brown. Add the garlic, jalapenos, red pepper flakes, and cumin. Cook for 3 minutes.
2. Add the lentils and stir in water, salt, and turmeric. Cover and cook on high within 2 hours and 30 minutes. Add spinach and mix. Cook on high for 15 minutes more. Serve.

Nutrition:

Calories: 280

Carbs: 49g

Fat: 2g

Protein: 21g

Bourbon Baked Beans

Preparation time: 15 minutes

Cooking time: 6 hours

Servings: 4 people

Ingredients:

- 1 large sweet onion, peeled and diced
- 3 (15-ounce) cans cannellini beans
- 1 (15-ounce) can diced tomatoes
- ¼ cup maple syrup
- 3 tbsp apple cider vinegar
- 1 tsp liquid smoke
- 4 cloves garlic, peeled and minced
- 2 tbsp dry mustard
- 1½ tsp ground black pepper
- ½ tsp ground ginger
- ¼ tsp dried red pepper flakes
- 2 tbsp bourbon

- Salt, to taste

Directions:

1. Add all the fixings to the slow cooker and mix. Cover and cook on low within 6 hours. Serve.

Nutrition:

Calories: 290

Carbs: 48g

Fat: 2g

Protein: 15g

Italian Chickpeas

Preparation time: 15 minutes

Cooking time: 4-6 hours

Servings: 4 people

Ingredients:

- 1-pound dry chickpeas, soaked overnight
- 1 (28-ounce) can no-salt-added diced tomatoes
- 1 onion, chopped
- 1 bell pepper, seeded and chopped
- 3 garlic cloves, minced
- 1 teaspoon salt
- ½ teaspoon freshly ground black pepper
- ½ teaspoon paprika
- ½ teaspoon dried basil
- ½ teaspoon dried oregano
- ½ teaspoon dried parsley
- ¼ teaspoon red pepper flakes

Directions:

1. Mix the chickpeas, tomatoes and their juices, onion, bell pepper, garlic, salt, pepper, paprika, basil, oregano, parsley, and red pepper flakes in the slow cooker. Stir to mix well.
2. Cook on low within 4 to 6 hours, or until the chickpeas are tender, and serve.

Nutrition:

Calories: 289

Fat: 5g

Carbs: 49g

Protein: 15g

Sweet and Spicy Chickpeas

Preparation time: 15 minutes

Cooking time: 4-6 hours

Servings: 4 people

Ingredients:

- 2 pounds dry chickpeas, soaked overnight
- 2 bell peppers, seeded and chopped
- 1 onion, chopped
- 1-pound potatoes, peeled and chopped
- ¾ cup honey
- 1/3 cup sriracha sauce
- 2 tablespoons low-sodium soy sauce or tamari
- 2 garlic cloves, minced
- 1 teaspoon dried basil

Directions:

1. In the slow cooker, combine the chickpeas, bell peppers, onion, and potatoes.
2. In a medium bowl, mix the honey, sriracha, soy sauce, garlic, and basil. Put the sauce into the slow cooker, then stir to combine well. Cook on low for 4 to 6 hours and serve.

Nutrition:

Calories: 570

Fat: 7g

Carbs: 109g

Protein: 24g

Mediterranean Chickpeas and Brown Rice

Preparation time: 15 minutes

Cooking time: 4-6 hours

Servings: 4 people

Ingredients:

- Nonstick cooking spray
- 1 (15-ounce) can chickpeas, drained and rinsed
- 1 cup uncooked brown rice
- 2½ cups low-sodium vegetable broth
- 3 garlic cloves, minced
- Juice of 1 lemon
- 1 tablespoon extra-virgin olive oil
- 1 teaspoon dried oregano
- 1 teaspoon paprika
- 1 teaspoon ground coriander

- 1 teaspoon ground cumin
- 1 teaspoon curry powder
- 1 teaspoon chili powder
- ½ teaspoon salt
- ¼ teaspoon freshly ground black pepper

Directions:

1. Oiled slow cooker generously with nonstick cooking spray. In the slow cooker, combine the chickpeas, rice, broth, garlic, lemon juice, olive oil, oregano, paprika, coriander, cumin, curry powder, chili powder, salt, and pepper.
2. Stir to mix well. Cook on low within 4 to 6 hours, or until the rice is tender, and serve.

Nutrition: Calories: 372 Fat: 8g Carbs: 62g Protein: 14g

Rice Pilaf

Preparation time: 15 minutes

Cooking time: 4-6 hours

Servings: 4 people

Ingredients:

- Nonstick cooking spray
- 1 cup uncooked long-grain brown rice
- 2¼ cups low-sodium vegetable broth
- 1 teaspoon extra-virgin olive oil
- ½ teaspoon salt
- 1/8 teaspoon freshly ground black pepper

Directions:

1. Oiled slow cooker generously with nonstick cooking spray. In the slow cooker, combine the rice, broth, olive oil, salt, and pepper. Stir to mix well. Cook on low within 4 to 6 hours and serve.

Nutrition: Calories: 203 Fat: 3g Carbs: 37g Protein: 6g

Wild Rice and Mushroom Casserole

Preparation time: 15 minutes

Cooking time: 5-7 hours

Servings: 4 people

Ingredients:

- Nonstick cooking spray
- 1-pound mushrooms, sliced
- ¾ cup uncooked wild rice
- 1½ cups low-sodium chicken broth
- 1 onion, finely chopped
- ¼ teaspoon dried thyme
- ¼ teaspoon dried basil
- ½ teaspoon salt
- ½ teaspoon freshly ground black pepper

- 2 tablespoons chopped fresh parsley

Directions:

1. Oiled slow cooker generously with nonstick cooking spray. In the slow cooker, combine the mushrooms, rice, broth, onion, thyme, basil, salt, and pepper. Stir to mix well.
2. Cook on low within 5 to 7 hours, or until the rice is tender. Top with fresh parsley and serve.

Nutrition:

Calories: 154

Fat: 1g

Carbs: 29g

Protein: 10g

Rice with Chicken and Asparagus

Preparation time: 15 minutes

Cooking time: 5-7 hours

Servings: 4 people

Ingredients:

- Nonstick cooking spray
- 1-pound boneless, skinless chicken breasts or thighs
- 1 cup uncooked brown rice
- 2½ cups water
- 1-pound asparagus, cut into 1-inch pieces
- 2 garlic cloves, minced
- Juice of 2 limes
- 1 teaspoon ground cumin
- ½ teaspoon salt
- ½ teaspoon freshly ground black pepper

Directions:

1. Oiled slow cooker generously with nonstick cooking spray. Mix the chicken, rice, water, asparagus, garlic, lime juice, cumin, salt, and pepper in the slow cooker. Stir to mix well. Cook on low within 5 to 7 hours, or until the rice is tender, and serve.

Nutrition:

Calories: 321

Fat: 3g

Carbs: 41g

Protein: 32g

Cilantro-Lime Chicken and Rice

Preparation time: 15 minutes

Cooking time: 5-7 hours

Servings: 4 people

Ingredients:

- Nonstick cooking spray
- 1-pound boneless, skinless chicken breasts or thighs
- 2 cups uncooked brown rice
- 4 cups of water
- 1 can no-salt-added diced tomatoes
- 1 can black beans, drained and rinsed
- 1 can corn, drained and rinsed
- 2 garlic cloves, minced
- Juice of 2 limes
- 1 teaspoon ground cumin
- 1 teaspoon salt
- ½ teaspoon freshly ground black pepper

- ½ teaspoon dried oregano
- ½ cup chopped fresh cilantro

Directions:

1. Oiled slow cooker generously with nonstick cooking spray. Mix the chicken, rice, water, tomatoes, beans, corn, garlic, lime juice, cumin, salt, pepper, and oregano in the slow cooker.
2. Stir to mix well. Cook on low within 5 to 7 hours, or until the rice is tender. Sprinkle with fresh cilantro before serving.

Nutrition:

Calories: 432

Fat: 3g

Carbs: 72g

Protein: 29g

Indian Spiced Brown Rice with Ground Lamb

Preparation time: 15 minutes

Cooking time: 4-6 hours

Servings: 4 people

Ingredients:

- 1 cup uncooked brown rice
- 2 cups low-sodium chicken broth
- 1 cup Marinara Sauce
- 1 onion, chopped
- 3 garlic cloves, minced
- 2 teaspoons curry powder or garam masala
- 2 teaspoons ground cumin
- 2 teaspoons ground ginger
- 2 teaspoons ground turmeric
- 1 teaspoon ground coriander

- ½ teaspoon ground cayenne pepper
- 1-pound ground lamb, cooked

Directions:

1. In the slow cooker, combine the rice, broth, marinara sauce, onion, garlic, curry powder, cumin, ginger, turmeric, coriander, and cayenne pepper. Stir to mix well. Cook on low within 4 to 6 hours. Stir in the ground lamb and serve.

Nutrition:

Calories: 325

Fat: 13g

Carbs: 33g

Protein: 18g

Barley and Chickpea Risotto

Preparation time: 15 minutes

Cooking time: 4-6 hours

Servings: 4 people

Ingredients:

- Nonstick cooking spray
- 1½ cups uncooked barley, rinsed
- 1 (15-ounce) can chickpeas, drained and rinsed
- 3 cups of water
- 2 garlic cloves, minced
- 1 onion, minced
- 1 teaspoon salt
- ½ teaspoon dried rosemary
- ½ teaspoon freshly ground black pepper
- ¼ cup grated Parmesan cheese
- ¼ cup chopped fresh parsley

Directions:

1. Oiled slow cooker generously with nonstick cooking spray. In the slow cooker, combine the barley, chickpeas, water, garlic, onion, salt, rosemary, pepper, and cheese. Stir to mix well. Cook on low within 4 to 6 hours. Top with fresh parsley before serving.

Tip: For more flavor, use low-sodium broth instead of water or a combo of the two.

Nutrition:

Calories: 445

Fat: 5g

Carbs: 83g

Protein: 17g

Coconut Quinoa Curry

Preparation time: 15 minutes

Cooking time: 6-8 hours

Servings: 4 people

Ingredients:

- 1 can full-fat coconut milk
- 1 cup Coconut-Curry Sauce
- 1 can no-salt-added diced tomatoes
- 1 cup uncooked quinoa, rinsed
- 1 small onion, chopped
- 2 garlic cloves, minced
- 1 tablespoon soy sauce
- 2 teaspoons curry powder
- 1 teaspoon ground ginger
- ½ teaspoon salt
- ½ teaspoon freshly ground black pepper
- ¼ teaspoon red pepper flakes

Directions:

1. In the slow cooker, combine the coconut milk, curry sauce, tomatoes, and their juices, quinoa, onion, garlic, soy sauce, curry powder, ginger, salt, pepper, and red pepper flakes. Stir to mix well. Cook on low within 6 to 8 hours and serve.

Nutrition:

Calories: 415

Fat: 32g

Carbs: 28g

Protein: 9g

Sweet and Sour Beans

Preparation time: 15 minutes

Cooking time: 7-8 hours & 15 minutes

Servings: 4 people

Ingredients:

- 1-pound white beans, soaked overnight
- 4 cups Vegetable Broth
- 1 can no-salt-added tomato paste
- 1 cup of water
- 3 carrots, diced
- 1 sweet onion, diced
- 2 bell peppers (red, orange, yellow, or green), diced
- ¼ cup Ketchup
- ¼ cup dry cooking sherry
- ¼ cup low-sodium tamari
- ¼ cup cider vinegar
- 2 tablespoons sugar

- 1 tablespoon dried marjoram
- 1 tablespoon dried thyme
- 2 teaspoons freshly ground black pepper
- 1 tablespoon cornstarch or arrowroot

Directions:

1. Drain and rinse the beans. Put them in a 6-quart slow cooker along with the broth, tomato paste, water, carrots, onion, bell peppers, ketchup, sherry, tamari, vinegar, sugar, marjoram, thyme, and pepper.
2. Cover and cook on low within 7 to 8 hours. With 15 minutes left before serving, stir in the cornstarch. Cook again within 15 minutes until the broth thickens. Serve warm.

Nutrition: Calories: 263 Fat: 0g Carbs: 49g Protein: 16g

Navy Bean Soup with Ham

Preparation time: 10 minutes

Cooking time: 8-10 hours

Servings: 4 people

Ingredients:

- 1-pound dried navy beans, drained & rinsed
- 2 cups Chicken Stock
- 1 can no-salt-added diced tomatoes
- 8 oz. 98% fat-free, reduced-sodium ham, finely diced
- 3 celery ribs, diced
- 3 carrots, diced
- 1 onion, diced
- 3 garlic cloves, minced
- 1½ teaspoons onion powder
- 1 teaspoon dried parsley
- 1 teaspoon dried sage

- 1 teaspoon garlic powder
- 1 bay leaf
- ½ teaspoon freshly ground black pepper
- ½ teaspoon salt

Directions:

1. Soak or dip the beans overnight at room temperature in a large bowl with 2 quarts of water. Put the beans in a 4- to 6-quart slow cooker.
2. Cover the beans with about 1 inch of water and add the rest of the ingredients. Stir well. Cover and cook on low within 8 to 10 hours.
3. Use the back of a spoon to mash some of the beans against the slow cooker's sides, then mix them back into the soup, creating a creamier texture. Serve hot.

Nutrition: Calories: 256 Fat: 0g Carbs: 44g Protein: 21g

Coconut Red Beans and Rice

Preparation time: 15 minutes

Cooking time: 7-8 hours

Servings: 4 people

Ingredients:

- 1 cup dried red beans, soaked overnight
- 4 cups Chicken Stock
- 1 can light coconut milk
- 1½ cups long-grain basmati white rice
- 1 large onion, finely diced
- 2 garlic cloves, minced
- 1 teaspoon red pepper flakes
- ½ teaspoon coconut extract (optional)
- 1-2 tablespoons squeezed lime juice
- 2 limes, cut into wedges, for serving

Directions:

1. Drain and rinse the soaked beans. Add the beans to a 6-quart slow cooker along with the stock, coconut milk, rice, onion, garlic, red pepper flakes, and coconut extract (if using). Stir well.
2. Cover and cook for 7 to 8 hours on low. Stir in the lime juice and taste to adjust seasonings. Serve warm, with the lime wedges on the side.

Nutrition:

Calories: 262

Fat: 2g

Carbs: 65g

Protein: 16g

Ranch Style Pinto Beans

Preparation time: 10 minutes

Cooking time: 7-8 hours

Servings: 4 people

Ingredients:

- 1-pound dried pinto beans, soaked overnight
- 5 cups Beef Stock
- 1 cup low-sodium tomato sauce
- 1 medium white onion, diced
- 1 jalapeño pepper, seeded and finely diced
- 4 garlic cloves, minced
- 1 tablespoon ancho chili powder
- 1 teaspoon chili powder
- 1 teaspoon apple cider vinegar
- 1 teaspoon ground cumin
- 1 packed teaspoon brown sugar
- 1 teaspoon smoked paprika

- ½ teaspoon dried oregano
- Freshly ground black pepper

Directions:

1. Drain and rinse the soaked beans. Put them in a 6-quart slow cooker along with the stock, tomato sauce, onion, jalapeño, garlic, ancho chili powder, chili powder, vinegar, cumin, sugar, paprika, and oregano.
2. Cover and cook on low within 7 to 8 hours, until the beans are tender and the liquid has thickened slightly—taste and season with the pepper. Serve warm.

Nutrition: Calories: 222 Fat: 0g Carbs: 40g Protein: 14g

Garlic Veggie Lentils

Preparation time: 15 minutes

Cooking time: 7-8 hours

Servings: 4 people

Ingredients:

- 3 cups dried lentils
- 5 cups Vegetable Broth
- 1 can no-salt-added diced tomatoes
- 1 large onion, chopped
- 2 leeks, chopped
- 8 garlic cloves, minced
- 2 large carrots, chopped
- 2 bay leaves
- 1 teaspoon dried thyme
- Freshly ground black pepper

Directions:

1. Sort the lentils, discarding any stones or impurities. Rinse under cold water in a fine-mesh strainer. Combine all of the ingredients in a 6-quart slow cooker and stir.
2. Cover and cook on low within 7 to 8 hours until the lentils are tender and the sauce has thickened. Remove and discard the bay leaf. Serve warm.

Nutrition:

Calories: 185

Fat: 0g

Carbs: 34g

Protein: 11g

Vegetarian Calico Beans

Preparation time: 15 minutes

Cooking time: 7-8 hours

Servings: 4 people

Ingredients:

- 6 cups Vegetable Broth
- 1 can lima beans, drained and rinsed
- 1 can fire-roasted tomatoes
- 1 cup dried kidney beans, soaked overnight
- 1 cup dried pinto beans, soaked overnight
- 1 large sweet onion, chopped
- 1 medium red bell pepper, chopped
- ½ cup Ketchup
- 1/3 cup loosely packed brown sugar
- 1 tablespoon Dijon mustard
- 1 tablespoon apple cider vinegar
- Freshly ground black pepper

Directions:

1. Combine the ingredients in a 6-quart slow cooker. Cover and cook on low within 7 to 8 hours, until the beans are tender. Serve warm.

Nutrition:

Calories: 246

Fat: 0g

Carbs: 47g

Protein: 13g

Summer Squash Mix

Preparation time: 15 minutes

Cooking time: 2 hours

Servings: 4 people

Ingredients:

- ¼ cup olive oil
- 2 tablespoons basil, chopped
- 2 tablespoons balsamic vinegar
- 2 garlic cloves, minced
- 2 teaspoons mustard
- Salt and black pepper to the taste
- 3 summer squash, sliced
- 2 zucchinis, sliced

Directions:

1. In your slow cooker, mix squash with zucchinis, salt, pepper, mustard, garlic, vinegar, basil, and oil, toss a bit, cook on high within 2 hours. Divide between plates and serve as a side dish.

Nutrition:

Calories: 179

Fat: 13g

Carbs: 10g

Protein: 4g

Hot Zucchini Mix

Preparation time: 5 minutes

Cooking time: 2 hours

Servings: 2 people

Ingredients:

- ¼ cup carrots, grated
- 1-pound zucchinis, roughly cubed
- 1 teaspoon hot paprika
- ½ teaspoon chili powder
- 2 spring onions, chopped
- ½ tablespoon olive oil
- ½ teaspoon curry powder
- 1 garlic clove, minced
- ½ teaspoon ginger powder
- A pinch of salt and black pepper
- 1 tablespoon cilantro, chopped

Directions:

1. In your slow cooker, mix the carrots with the zucchinis, paprika, and the rest of the fixing, toss, cook on low for 2 hours. Divide between plates and serve as a side dish.

Nutrition:

Calories: 200

Fat: 5g

Carbs: 28g

Protein: 4g

Creamy Butter Parsnips

Preparation time: 15 minutes

Cooking time: 7 hours

Servings: 4 people

Ingredients:

- 1 cup cream
- 2 tsp butter
- 1 lb. parsnip, peeled and chopped
- 1 carrot, chopped
- 1 yellow onion, chopped
- 1 tbsp chives, chopped
- 1 tsp salt
- 1 tsp ground white pepper
- ½ tsp paprika
- 1 tbsp salt
- ¼ tsp sugar

Directions:

1. Add parsnips, carrots, and the rest of the ingredients to the slow cooker. Put the cooker's lid on and set the cooking time to 7 hours on low. Serve warm.

Nutrition:

Calories: 190

Fat: 11.2g

Carbs: 22g

Protein: 3g

Butternut Squash and Eggplant Mix

Preparation time: 15 minutes

Cooking time: 4 hours

Servings: 2 people

Ingredients:

- 1 butternut squash, peeled and roughly cubed
- 1 eggplant, roughly cubed
- 1 red onion, chopped
- Cooking spray
- ½ cup veggie stock
- ¼ cup tomato paste
- ½ tablespoon parsley, chopped
- Salt and black pepper to the taste
- 2 garlic cloves, minced

Directions:

1. Grease the slow cooker with the cooking spray and mix the squash with the eggplant, onion, and the other ingredients inside.
2. Cook on low within 4 hours. Divide between plates and serve as a side dish. it

Nutrition:

Calories: 114

Fat: 4g

Carbs: 18g

Protein: 4g

Classic Veggies Mix

Preparation time: 15 minutes

Cooking time: 3 hours

Servings: 4 people

Ingredients:

- 1 and ½ cups red onion, cut into medium chunks
- 1 cup cherry tomatoes, halved
- 2 and ½ cups zucchini, sliced
- 2 cups yellow bell pepper, chopped
- 1 cup mushrooms, sliced
- 2 tablespoons basil, chopped
- 1 tablespoon thyme, chopped
- ½ cup olive oil
- ½ cup balsamic vinegar

Directions:

1. In your slow cooker, mix onion pieces with tomatoes, zucchini, bell pepper, mushrooms, basil, thyme, oil,

and vinegar, toss to coat everything, cover, and cook on high for 3 hours. Divide between plates and serve as a side dish.

Nutrition:

Calories: 150

Fat: 2g

Carbs: 6g

Protein: 5g

Spinach and Squash Side Salad

Preparation time: 15 minutes

Cooking time: 4 hours

Servings: 4 people

Ingredients:

- 3 pounds butternut squash, peeled and cubed
- 1 yellow onion, chopped
- 2 teaspoons thyme, chopped
- 3 garlic cloves, minced
- A pinch of salt and black pepper
- 10 oz. veggie stock
- 6 oz. baby spinach

Directions:

1. In your slow cooker, mix squash cubes with onion, thyme, salt, pepper, and stock, stir, cover, and cook on low for 4 hours. Transfer squash mixture to a bowl, add spinach, toss, divide between plates and serve as a side dish.

Nutrition:

Calories: 100

Fat: 1g

Carbs: 18g

Protein: 4g

Cheddar Potatoes Mix

Preparation time: 15 minutes

Cooking time: 3 hours

Servings: 2 people

Ingredients:

- ½ pound gold potatoes, cut into wedges
- 2 oz. heavy cream
- ½ teaspoon turmeric powder
- ½ teaspoon rosemary, dried
- ¼ cup cheddar cheese, shredded
- 1 tablespoon butter, melted
- Cooking spray
- A pinch of salt and black pepper

Directions:

1. Grease your slow cooker with the cooking spray, add the potatoes, cream, turmeric, and the rest of the

fixing, toss, put the lid on and cook on high for 3 hours. Divide between plates and serve as a side dish.

Nutrition:

Calories: 300

Fat: 14g

Carbs: 22g

Protein: 6g

Okra and Corn

Preparation time: 15 minutes

Cooking time: 8 hours

Servings: 4 people

Ingredients:

- 3 garlic cloves, minced
- 1 small green bell pepper, chopped
- 1 small yellow onion, chopped
- 1 cup of water
- 16 oz. okra, sliced
- 2 cups corn
- 1 and ½ teaspoon smoked paprika
- 28 oz. canned tomatoes, crushed
- 1 teaspoon oregano, dried
- 1 teaspoon thyme, dried
- 1 teaspoon marjoram, dried
- A pinch of cayenne pepper

- Salt and black pepper to the taste

Directions:

1. In your slow cooker, mix garlic with bell pepper, onion, water, okra, corn, paprika, tomatoes, oregano, thyme, marjoram, cayenne, salt and pepper, cover, cook on low for 8 hours, divide between plates and serve as a side dish.

Nutrition:

Calories: 182

Fat: 3g

Carbs: 8g

Protein: 5g

www.ingramcontent.com/pod-product-compliance
Lightning Source LLC
Chambersburg PA
CBHW071112030426
42336CB00013BA/2049